PRE-DIABETES DIET PLAN AND RECIPE BOOK

30-Day Meal Plan & Delicious Recipes for Balanced Blood Sugar

T. John

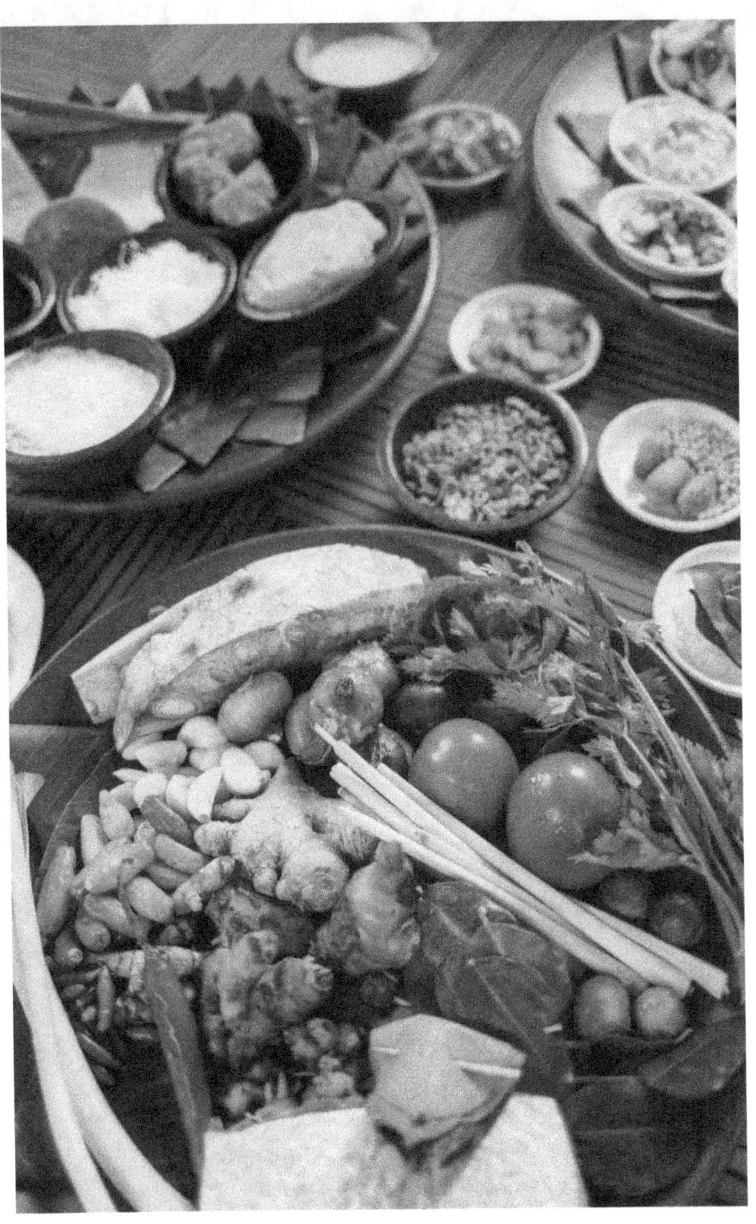

TABLE OF CONTENTS

Chapter 3: Lunch Recipes..41

Chapter 4: Dinner Recipes 60

INTRODUCTION

I magine your body's response to sugar is like a see-saw. Normally, insulin, a hormone, acts like a counterweight, keeping blood sugar levels balanced. But in pre-diabetes, the see-saw gets stuck. Your body produces insulin, but it's not as effective, causing blood sugar to rise. This is where diet steps in, becoming your powerful tool to manage pre-diabetes and potentially prevent it from progressing to type 2 diabetes.

Understanding the Power of Plate:

Think of your plate as a blueprint for managing blood sugar. Here's how different food groups play their roles:

- **Non-starchy Vegetables**: These champions are low in calories and carbohydrates, providing essential vitamins and fiber. Pile on the leafy greens, broccoli, cauliflower, and peppers!
- **Whole Grains**: Opt for brown rice, quinoa, oats, and whole-wheat bread over their refined counterparts.

They release sugar slowly, preventing blood sugar spikes.

- **Lean Protein**: Chicken, fish, beans, and lentils offer sustained energy without excessive saturated fat.
- **Healthy Fats**: Include moderate amounts of avocados, nuts, and olive oil for satiety and heart health.
- **Fruits**: Enjoy them in moderation, choosing low-glycemic varieties like berries and apples.
- **Limit**: Added sugars, sugary drinks, refined grains, and unhealthy fats are the villains in this story. Minimize them to keep your blood sugar in check.

Tips for Dietary Success:

- **Small, frequent meals**: Instead of 3 large meals, spread your food intake across 5-6 smaller portions throughout the day. This helps maintain stable blood sugar levels.
- **Fiber is your friend**: Aim for 25-30 grams of fiber daily. It slows down digestion, promoting satiety and regulating blood sugar.

- **Read food labels**: Be mindful of hidden sugars and serving sizes. Opt for whole, unprocessed foods whenever possible.

- **Spice it up!:** Experiment with herbs and spices to add flavor without added sodium or sugars.

- **Plan and prep**: Planning meals and prepping healthy snacks in advance will help you resist unhealthy temptations.

- **Don't go it alone**: Seek support from a registered dietitian or nutritionist for personalized guidance.

Remember:

- **Consistency is key**: Making small, sustainable changes over time is more effective than drastic short-term efforts.

- **Celebrate progress**: Every healthy choice is a victory. Acknowledge your wins to stay motivated.

- **Enjoy the journey**: Explore new recipes, discover delicious healthy options, and make mealtimes a source of joy, not restriction.

By understanding the role of diet and incorporating these tips, you can empower yourself to manage pre-diabetes and pave the way for a healthier future. Remember, you are not alone in this journey. With the right knowledge and support, you can take control of your health and thrive!

Chapter 1: 30 Day Meal Plan

Week 1:

Day 1:

- Breakfast: Quinoa Breakfast Bowl
- Lunch: Grilled Chicken Salad with Balsamic Vinaigrette
- Dinner: Baked Lemon Herb Chicken
- Snack: Guacamole with Veggie Sticks
- Dessert: Mixed Berry Parfait

Day 2:

- Breakfast: Vegetable Omelette
- Lunch: Quinoa and Black Bean Bowl
- Dinner: Spaghetti Squash with Turkey Bolognese
- Snack: Hummus and Whole Wheat Pita
- Dessert: Dark Chocolate-Dipped Strawberries

Day 3:

- Breakfast: Greek Yogurt Parfait
- Lunch: Turkey and Vegetable Wrap

- Dinner: Grilled Vegetable and Quinoa Stuffed Bell Peppers
- Snack: Greek Yogurt with Berries
- Dessert: Greek Yogurt and Honey Popsicles

Day 4:

- Breakfast: Avocado Toast with Poached Egg
- Lunch: Lentil Soup
- Dinner: Teriyaki Salmon with Brown Rice
- Snack: Roasted Chickpeas
- Dessert: Baked Apple with Cinnamon

Day 5:

- Breakfast: Chia Seed Pudding with Berries
- Lunch: Salmon and Asparagus Foil Pack
- Dinner: Cauliflower Crust Margherita Pizza
- Snack: Cottage Cheese and Pineapple
- Dessert: Berry and Almond Crisp

Day 6:

- Breakfast: Spinach and Mushroom Frittata
- Lunch: Chickpea and Spinach Stew

- Dinner: Blackened Tilapia with Quinoa Pilaf

- Snack: Caprese Skewers

- Dessert: Avocado Chocolate Mousse

Day 7:

- Breakfast: Whole Grain Pancakes with Fruit Compote

- Lunch: Shrimp and Quinoa Stir-Fry

- Dinner: Turkey and Sweet Potato Skillet

- Snack: Trail Mix with Nuts and Dried Fruit

- Dessert: Pumpkin Pie Chia Pudding

Week 2:

Day 8:

- Breakfast: Overnight Oats with Almond Butter

- Lunch: Caprese Salad with Whole Grain Bread

- Dinner: Eggplant Lasagna

- Snack: Sliced Apple with Almond Butter

- Dessert: Coconut and Berry Sorbet

Day 9:

- Breakfast: Smoked Salmon and Cream Cheese Bagel

- Lunch: Turkey and Avocado Wrap

- Dinner: Coconut Curry Chicken with Vegetables

- Snack: Baked Sweet Potato Fries

- Dessert: Almond Flour Banana Bread

Day 10:

- Breakfast: Sweet Potato Hash with Turkey Sausage

- Lunch: Mediterranean Chickpea Salad

- Dinner: Lemon Garlic Shrimp with Whole Wheat Pasta

- Snack: Edamame with Sea Salt

- Dessert: Mango and Yogurt Frozen Bites

Day 11:

- Breakfast: Banana Walnut Muffins

- Lunch: Broccoli and Cheddar Stuffed Baked Potatoes

- Dinner: Stuffed Acorn Squash with Wild Rice

- Snack: Cucumber and Feta Bites

- Dessert: Chocolate Avocado Truffles

Day 12:

- Breakfast: Veggie and Cheese Breakfast Burrito
- Lunch: Vegetable and Tofu Stir-Fry
- Dinner: Ratatouille
- Snack: Greek Hummus Dip
- Dessert: Lemon Blueberry Yogurt Cake

Day 13:

- Breakfast: Berry Protein Smoothie Bowl
- Lunch: Greek Chicken Gyro
- Dinner: Sesame Ginger Tofu Stir-Fry
- Snack: Almond and Cranberry Energy Balls
- Dessert: Strawberry Shortcake Cups

Day 14:

- Breakfast: Almond Flour Waffles
- Lunch: Tomato Basil Soup with Whole Grain Croutons
- Dinner: Cilantro Lime Chicken with Brown Rice
- Snack: Salsa and Whole Grain Tortilla Chips
- Dessert: Pistachio and Cranberry Bark

Week 3:

Day 15:

- Breakfast: Egg and Veggie Breakfast Wrap
- Lunch: Zucchini Noodles with Pesto and Cherry Tomatoes
- Dinner: Roasted Brussels Sprouts and Chicken Thighs
- Snack: Stuffed Mini Bell Peppers with Goat Cheese
- Dessert: Raspberry and Almond Chia Seed Pudding

Day 16:

- Breakfast: Quinoa Breakfast Bowl
- Lunch: Grilled Chicken Salad with Balsamic Vinaigrette
- Dinner: Baked Lemon Herb Chicken
- Snack: Guacamole with Veggie Sticks
- Dessert: Mixed Berry Parfait

Day 17:

- Breakfast: Vegetable Omelette
- Lunch: Quinoa and Black Bean Bowl
- Dinner: Spaghetti Squash with Turkey Bolognese

- Snack: Hummus and Whole Wheat Pita
- Dessert: Dark Chocolate-Dipped Strawberries

Day 18:

- Breakfast: Greek Yogurt Parfait
- Lunch: Turkey and Vegetable Wrap
- Dinner: Grilled Vegetable and Quinoa Stuffed Bell Peppers
- Snack: Greek Yogurt with Berries
- Dessert: Greek Yogurt and Honey Popsicles

Day 19:

- Breakfast: Avocado Toast with Poached Egg
- Lunch: Lentil Soup
- Dinner: Teriyaki Salmon with Brown Rice
- Snack: Roasted Chickpeas
- Dessert: Baked Apple with Cinnamon

Day 20:

- Breakfast: Chia Seed Pudding with Berries
- Lunch: Salmon and Asparagus Foil Pack
- Dinner: Cauliflower Crust Margherita Pizza

- Snack: Cottage Cheese and Pineapple
- Dessert: Berry and Almond Crisp

Day 21:

- Breakfast: Spinach and Mushroom Frittata
- Lunch: Chickpea and Spinach Stew
- Dinner: Blackened Tilapia with Quinoa Pilaf
- Snack: Caprese Skewers
- Dessert: Avocado Chocolate Mousse

Week 4:

Day 22:

- Breakfast: Whole Grain Pancakes with Fruit Compote
- Lunch: Shrimp and Quinoa Stir-Fry
- Dinner: Turkey and Sweet Potato Skillet
- Snack: Trail Mix with Nuts and Dried Fruit
- Dessert: Pumpkin Pie Chia Pudding

Day 23:

- Breakfast: Overnight Oats with Almond Butter
- Lunch: Caprese Salad with Whole Grain Bread

- Dinner: Eggplant Lasagna
- Snack: Sliced Apple with Almond Butter
- Dessert: Coconut and Berry Sorbet

Day 24:

- Breakfast: Smoked Salmon and Cream Cheese Bagel
- Lunch: Turkey and Avocado Wrap
- Dinner: Coconut Curry Chicken with Vegetables
- Snack: Baked Sweet Potato Fries
- Dessert: Almond Flour Banana Bread

Day 25:

- Breakfast: Sweet Potato Hash with Turkey Sausage
- Lunch: Mediterranean Chickpea Salad
- Dinner: Lemon Garlic Shrimp with Whole Wheat Pasta
- Snack: Edamame with Sea Salt
- Dessert: Mango and Yogurt Frozen Bites

Day 26:

- Breakfast: Banana Walnut Muffins

- Lunch: Broccoli and Cheddar Stuffed Baked Potatoes
- Dinner: Stuffed Acorn Squash with Wild Rice
- Snack: Cucumber and Feta Bites
- Dessert: Chocolate Avocado Truffles

Day 27:

- Breakfast: Veggie and Cheese Breakfast Burrito
- Lunch: Vegetable and Tofu Stir-Fry
- Dinner: Ratatouille
- Snack: Greek Hummus Dip
- Dessert: Lemon Blueberry Yogurt Cake

Day 28:

- Breakfast: Berry Protein Smoothie Bowl
- Lunch: Greek Chicken Gyro
- Dinner: Sesame Ginger Tofu Stir-Fry
- Snack: Almond and Cranberry Energy Balls
- Dessert: Strawberry Shortcake Cups

Day 29:

- Breakfast: Almond Flour Waffles

- Lunch: Tomato Basil Soup with Whole Grain Croutons
- Dinner: Cilantro Lime Chicken with Brown Rice
- Snack: Salsa and Whole Grain Tortilla Chips
- Dessert: Pistachio and Cranberry Bark

Day 30:

- Breakfast: Egg and Veggie Breakfast Wrap
- Lunch: Zucchini Noodles with Pesto and Cherry Tomatoes
- Dinner: Roasted Brussels Sprouts and Chicken Thighs
- Snack: Stuffed Mini Bell Peppers with Goat Cheese
- Dessert: Raspberry and Almond Chia Seed Pudding

Chapter 2: Breakfast Recipes

Breakfast is a crucial meal, especially for those managing pre-diabetes. These recipes are thoughtfully crafted to provide a balance of essential nutrients, keeping you energized and supporting your well-being.

Quinoa Breakfast Bowl:

Ingredients:

- 1 cup cooked quinoa
- 1/2 cup mixed berries
- 1 tablespoon honey
- 2 tablespoons chopped nuts (almonds, walnuts)

Instructions:

1. In a bowl, combine cooked quinoa and mixed berries.
2. Drizzle honey over the mixture.
3. Top with chopped nuts.
4. Stir gently and enjoy!

Nutrition Information:

- Calories: 300
- Protein: 8g
- Carbohydrates: 50g
- Fat: 7g
- Fiber: 6g
- Sugar: 15g
- Portion Size: 1 serving

Vegetable Omelette:

Ingredients:

- 2 eggs
- 1/4 cup diced bell peppers (mixed colors)
- 1/4 cup diced tomatoes
- 1/4 cup chopped spinach
- Salt and pepper to taste

Instructions:

1. Whisk eggs in a bowl and season with salt and pepper.
2. Pour the egg mixture into a heated, oiled pan.
3. Add vegetables on one half of the omelette.

4. Fold the omelette and cook until eggs are set.

Nutrition Information:

- Calories: 180
- Protein: 14g
- Carbohydrates: 6g
- Fat: 12g
- Fiber: 2g
- Sugar: 3g
- Portion Size: 1 serving

Greek Yogurt Parfait:

Ingredients:

- 1 cup Greek yogurt
- 1/2 cup granola
- 1/2 cup mixed berries
- 1 tablespoon honey

Instructions:

1. In a glass, layer Greek yogurt, granola, and mixed berries.
2. Drizzle honey over the top.

3. Repeat layers until the glass is filled.

4. Enjoy the parfait with a long spoon!

Nutrition Information:

- Calories: 320
- Protein: 18g
- Carbohydrates: 45g
- Fat: 8g
- Fiber: 6g
- Sugar: 20g
- Portion Size: 1 serving

Avocado Toast with Poached Egg:

Ingredients:

- 1 slice whole-grain bread
- 1/2 ripe avocado
- 1 poached egg
- Salt and pepper to taste

Instructions:

1. Toast the bread slice.

2. Mash the ripe avocado and spread it over the toast.

3. Top with a poached egg.

4. Season with salt and pepper.

Nutrition Information:

- Calories: 250
- Protein: 12g
- Carbohydrates: 20g
- Fat: 15g
- Fiber: 7g
- Sugar: 2g
- Portion Size: 1 serving

Chia Seed Pudding with Berries:

Ingredients:

- 2 tablespoons chia seeds
- 1 cup unsweetened almond milk
- 1/2 cup mixed berries
- 1 teaspoon honey

Instructions:

1. Mix chia seeds and almond milk in a jar.

2. Refrigerate overnight.

3. In the morning, layer chia pudding with mixed berries.

4. Drizzle honey on top.

Nutrition Information:

- Calories: 180

- Protein: 5g

- Carbohydrates: 25g

- Fat: 8g

- Fiber: 10g

- Sugar: 8g

- Portion Size: 1 serving

Spinach and Mushroom Frittata:

Ingredients:

- 4 eggs

- 1 cup fresh spinach

- 1/2 cup sliced mushrooms

- 1/4 cup feta cheese

- Salt and pepper to taste

Instructions:

1. Preheat oven to 375°F (190°C).
2. Whisk eggs and season with salt and pepper.
3. Sauté spinach and mushrooms in an oven-safe pan.
4. Pour whisked eggs over the veggies, add feta, and bake until set.

Nutrition Information:

- Calories: 220
- Protein: 18g
- Carbohydrates: 4g
- Fat: 15g
- Fiber: 2g
- Sugar: 1g
- Portion Size: 1 serving

Whole Grain Pancakes with Fruit Compote:

Ingredients:

- 1 cup whole wheat flour
- 1 tablespoon baking powder

- 1 cup almond milk

- 1 tablespoon maple syrup

- Mixed fruit compote (berries, peaches)

Instructions:

1. Mix flour, baking powder, almond milk, and maple syrup.

2. Cook pancakes on a griddle.

3. Top with mixed fruit compote.

Nutrition Information:

- Calories: 280

- Protein: 8g

- Carbohydrates: 45g

- Fat: 6g

- Fiber: 7g

- Sugar: 12g

- Portion Size: 2 pancakes

Overnight Oats with Almond Butter:

Ingredients:

- 1/2 cup rolled oats

- 1/2 cup unsweetened almond milk
- 1 tablespoon almond butter
- 1 tablespoon chia seeds
- Sliced banana for topping

Instructions:

1. Mix oats, almond milk, almond butter, and chia seeds in a jar.
2. Refrigerate overnight.
3. In the morning, stir well and top with sliced banana.

Nutrition Information:

- Calories: 300
- Protein: 10g
- Carbohydrates: 40g
- Fat: 12g
- Fiber: 8g
- Sugar: 6g
- Portion Size: 1 serving

Smoked Salmon and Cream Cheese Bagel:

Ingredients:

- 1 whole grain bagel
- 2 tablespoons light cream cheese
- 2 ounces smoked salmon
- Sliced cucumber and red onion

Instructions:

1. Toast the bagel.
2. Spread cream cheese on each half.
3. Layer with smoked salmon, cucumber, and red onion slices.

Nutrition Information:

- Calories: 350
- Protein: 20g
- Carbohydrates: 45g
- Fat: 12g
- Fiber: 6g
- Sugar: 5g
- Portion Size: 1 serving

Sweet Potato Hash with Turkey Sausage:

Ingredients:

- 1 medium sweet potato, diced
- 1/2 cup lean ground turkey sausage
- 1/4 cup diced bell peppers
- 1/4 cup diced onions
- 1 teaspoon olive oil

Instructions:

1. In a pan, sauté sweet potatoes, turkey sausage, bell peppers, and onions in olive oil until cooked.
2. Season with salt and pepper.

Nutrition Information:

- Calories: 280
- Protein: 15g
- Carbohydrates: 35g
- Fat: 10g
- Fiber: 6g
- Sugar: 8g
- Portion Size: 1 serving

Banana Walnut Muffins:

Ingredients:

- 1 cup whole wheat flour
- 1/2 cup mashed ripe bananas
- 1/4 cup chopped walnuts
- 1/4 cup honey
- 1/4 cup plain Greek yogurt
- 1 teaspoon baking powder

Instructions:

1. Preheat the oven to 350°F (175°C).
2. In a bowl, mix flour, mashed bananas, walnuts, honey, Greek yogurt, and baking powder.
3. Spoon the batter into muffin cups.
4. Bake for 20-25 minutes or until a toothpick comes out clean.

Nutrition Information:

- Calories: 180
- Protein: 5g
- Carbohydrates: 30g
- Fat: 6g

- Fiber: 3g
- Sugar: 15g
- Portion Size: 1 muffin

Veggie and Cheese Breakfast Burrito:

Ingredients:

- 1 whole grain tortilla
- 2 eggs, scrambled
- 1/4 cup diced bell peppers
- 1/4 cup diced tomatoes
- 1/4 cup shredded cheese
- Salsa for topping

Instructions:

1. In a heated skillet, cook scrambled eggs with bell peppers and tomatoes.
2. Place the egg mixture on a tortilla.
3. Add shredded cheese and roll into a burrito.
4. Top with salsa.

Nutrition Information:

- Calories: 320
- Protein: 18g
- Carbohydrates: 25g
- Fat: 16g
- Fiber: 5g
- Sugar: 3g
- Portion Size: 1 burrito

Berry Protein Smoothie Bowl:

Ingredients:

- 1 cup mixed berries (strawberries, blueberries, raspberries)
- 1/2 cup plain Greek yogurt
- 1 scoop vanilla protein powder
- 1/4 cup almond milk
- Toppings: granola, chia seeds, sliced almonds

Instructions:

1. Blend mixed berries, Greek yogurt, protein powder, and almond milk until smooth.
2. Pour into a bowl and add your favorite toppings.

Nutrition Information:

- Calories: 280
- Protein: 25g
- Carbohydrates: 30g
- Fat: 8g
- Fiber: 7g
- Sugar: 15g
- Portion Size: 1 serving

Almond Flour Waffles:

Ingredients:

- 1 cup almond flour
- 2 eggs
- 1/4 cup almond milk
- 1 tablespoon honey
- 1/2 teaspoon baking powder

Instructions:

1. Preheat the waffle maker.
2. In a bowl, mix almond flour, eggs, almond milk, honey, and baking powder.

3. Pour the batter into the waffle maker and cook according to the manufacturer's instructions.

Nutrition Information:

- Calories: 220
- Protein: 10g
- Carbohydrates: 15g
- Fat: 15g
- Fiber: 3g
- Sugar: 6g
- Portion Size: 2 waffles

Egg and Veggie Breakfast Wrap:

Ingredients:

- 1 whole grain tortilla
- 2 eggs, scrambled
- 1/4 cup diced bell peppers
- 1/4 cup diced tomatoes
- Handful of spinach
- Salt and pepper to taste

Instructions:

1. In a heated skillet, cook scrambled eggs with bell peppers, tomatoes, and spinach.

2. Place the egg mixture on a tortilla.

3. Season with salt and pepper, then wrap it up.

Nutrition Information:

- Calories: 280

- Protein: 15g

- Carbohydrates: 25g

- Fat: 12g

- Fiber: 5g

- Sugar: 3g

- Portion Size: 1 wrap

Chapter 3: Lunch Recipes

In this chapter, we've curated lunch recipes that are not only satisfying but also tailored to help you manage pre-diabetes. Each recipe features bold flavors and a careful balance of essential nutrients.

Grilled Chicken Salad with Balsamic Vinaigrette

Ingredients:

- 1 boneless, skinless chicken breast
- Mixed salad greens
- Cherry tomatoes, halved
- Cucumber, sliced
- Red onion, thinly sliced
- Balsamic vinaigrette dressing

Instructions:

1. Grill the chicken breast until fully cooked.
2. Slice the grilled chicken into strips.

3. In a large bowl, combine the salad greens, cherry tomatoes, cucumber, and red onion.

4. Top the salad with grilled chicken strips.

5. Drizzle balsamic vinaigrette over the salad and toss gently.

Nutrition Information:

- Calories: 350
- Protein: 25g
- Carbohydrates: 20g
- Fat: 18g
- Fiber: 5g
- Sugar: 8g
- Portion Size: 1 serving

Quinoa and Black Bean Bowl

Ingredients:

- 1 cup cooked quinoa
- 1 cup black beans, drained and rinsed
- Corn kernels
- Avocado, diced
- Fresh cilantro, chopped

- Lime juice

Instructions:

1. In a bowl, combine cooked quinoa, black beans, corn, avocado, and cilantro.
2. Squeeze lime juice over the mixture and toss gently.

Nutrition Information:

- Calories: 320
- Protein: 15g
- Carbohydrates: 45g
- Fat: 10g
- Fiber: 12g
- Sugar: 2g
- Portion Size: 1 serving

Turkey and Vegetable Wrap

Ingredients:

- Whole wheat wrap
- Turkey slices
- Hummus
- Spinach leaves

- Tomatoes, sliced
- Red bell pepper, thinly sliced

Instructions:

1. Spread hummus on the whole wheat wrap.
2. Layer turkey slices, spinach leaves, sliced tomatoes, and red bell pepper.
3. Roll the wrap tightly, cut in half, and secure with toothpicks.

Nutrition Information:

- Calories: 280
- Protein: 20g
- Carbohydrates: 30g
- Fat: 12g
- Fiber: 8g
- Sugar: 5g
- Portion Size: 1 serving

Lentil Soup

Ingredients:

- 1 cup dried lentils

- Vegetable broth

- Carrots, diced

- Celery, diced

- Onion, chopped

- Garlic, minced

- Cumin, ground

- Bay leaves

- Salt and pepper to taste

Instructions:

1. Rinse lentils and place them in a pot with vegetable broth.
2. Add carrots, celery, onion, garlic, cumin, bay leaves, salt, and pepper.
3. Simmer until lentils and vegetables are tender.

Nutrition Information:

- Calories: 220

- Protein: 18g

- Carbohydrates: 40g

- Fat: 1g

- Fiber: 16g

- Sugar: 4g

- Portion Size: 1 serving

Salmon and Asparagus Foil Pack

Ingredients:

- Salmon fillet

- Asparagus spears

- Lemon slices

- Olive oil

- Garlic, minced

- Dill, chopped

- Salt and pepper to taste

Instructions:

1. Preheat the oven to 400°F (200°C).

2. Place salmon fillet on a piece of foil.

3. Arrange asparagus around the salmon, add lemon slices, minced garlic, and sprinkle with dill.

4. Drizzle olive oil over the salmon and vegetables.

5. Seal the foil tightly and bake for 20-25 minutes.

Nutrition Information:

- Calories: 300
- Protein: 25g
- Carbohydrates: 8g
- Fat: 18g
- Fiber: 3g
- Sugar: 2g
- Portion Size: 1 serving

Chickpea and Spinach Stew

Ingredients:

- Chickpeas, cooked
- Fresh spinach
- Tomatoes, diced
- Onion, chopped
- Garlic, minced
- Vegetable broth
- Cumin, ground
- Paprika
- Salt and pepper to taste

Instructions:

1. In a pot, sauté onion and garlic until softened.
2. Add chickpeas, tomatoes, spinach, vegetable broth, cumin, paprika, salt, and pepper.
3. Simmer until spinach wilts and flavors meld.

Nutrition Information:

- Calories: 240
- Protein: 12g
- Carbohydrates: 38g
- Fat: 5g
- Fiber: 10g
- Sugar: 8g
- Portion Size: 1 serving

Shrimp and Quinoa Stir-Fry

Ingredients:

- Shrimp, peeled and deveined
- Quinoa, cooked
- Broccoli florets
- Bell peppers, sliced
- Soy sauce

- Sesame oil

- Ginger, grated

- Garlic, minced

- Green onions, sliced

Instructions:

1. In a wok, stir-fry shrimp, broccoli, and bell peppers in sesame oil.

2. Add cooked quinoa, soy sauce, ginger, and garlic.

3. Cook until shrimp are pink and vegetables are tender.

4. Garnish with sliced green onions.

Nutrition Information:

- Calories: 280

- Protein: 20g

- Carbohydrates: 30g

- Fat: 10g

- Fiber: 6g

- Sugar: 4g

- Portion Size: 1 serving

Caprese Salad with Whole Grain Bread

Ingredients:

- Cherry tomatoes, halved
- Fresh mozzarella, sliced
- Basil leaves
- Whole grain bread, toasted
- Balsamic glaze
- Olive oil
- Salt and pepper to taste

Instructions:

1. Arrange tomatoes, mozzarella, and basil on a plate.
2. Drizzle with balsamic glaze and olive oil.
3. Season with salt and pepper.
4. Serve with toasted whole grain bread.

Nutrition Information:

- Calories: 250
- Protein: 15g
- Carbohydrates: 25g
- Fat: 12g

- Fiber: 5g

- Sugar: 4g

- Portion Size: 1 serving

Turkey and Avocado Wrap

Ingredients:

- Whole wheat wrap

- Turkey slices

- Avocado, sliced

- Lettuce leaves

- Tomato, sliced

- Greek yogurt

- Lime juice

- Cilantro, chopped

Instructions:

1. Lay out the whole wheat wrap.

2. Layer turkey, avocado, lettuce, and tomato.

3. Mix Greek yogurt with lime juice and cilantro, spread on the wrap.

4. Roll tightly, cut in half, and secure with toothpicks.

Nutrition Information:

- Calories: 320
- Protein: 18g
- Carbohydrates: 30g
- Fat: 15g
- Fiber: 8g
- Sugar: 3g
- Portion Size: 1 serving

Mediterranean Chickpea Salad

Ingredients:

- Chickpeas, cooked
- Cherry tomatoes, halved
- Cucumber, diced
- Red onion, finely chopped
- Kalamata olives, sliced
- Feta cheese, crumbled
- Olive oil
- Lemon juice
- Oregano, dried
- Salt and pepper to taste

Instructions:

1. In a bowl, combine chickpeas, tomatoes, cucumber, red onion, olives, and feta.
2. Drizzle with olive oil and lemon juice.
3. Sprinkle with dried oregano, salt, and pepper.
4. Toss gently and serve.

Nutrition Information:

- Calories: 280
- Protein: 12g
- Carbohydrates: 30g
- Fat: 14g
- Fiber: 8g
- Sugar: 4g
- Portion Size: 1 serving

Broccoli and Cheddar Stuffed Baked Potatoes

Ingredients:

- Baking potatoes
- Broccoli florets, steamed

- Cheddar cheese, shredded

- Greek yogurt

- Green onions, sliced

- Salt and pepper to taste

Instructions:

1. Bake potatoes until tender.

2. Cut a slit in each potato and fluff the insides.

3. Fill with steamed broccoli, cheddar cheese, Greek yogurt, and green onions.

4. Season with salt and pepper.

Nutrition Information:

- Calories: 320

- Protein: 15g

- Carbohydrates: 45g

- Fat: 10g

- Fiber: 7g

- Sugar: 3g

- Portion Size: 1 serving

Vegetable and Tofu Stir-Fry

Ingredients:

- Firm tofu, cubed
- Broccoli florets
- Bell peppers, sliced
- Carrots, julienned
- Snow peas
- Soy sauce
- Sesame oil
- Ginger, grated
- Garlic, minced

Instructions:

1. Sauté tofu in sesame oil until golden.
2. Add broccoli, bell peppers, carrots, snow peas, ginger, and garlic.
3. Stir in soy sauce and cook until vegetables are tender.

Nutrition Information:

- Calories: 250
- Protein: 18g
- Carbohydrates: 20g

- Fat: 12g

- Fiber: 6g

- Sugar: 4g

- Portion Size: 1 serving

Greek Chicken Gyro

Ingredients:

- Chicken breast, grilled and sliced

- Whole wheat pita

- Tzatziki sauce

- Tomato, diced

- Red onion, thinly sliced

- Lettuce leaves

Instructions:

1. Warm the whole wheat pita.

2. Layer grilled chicken, tzatziki sauce, tomato, red onion, and lettuce.

3. Fold the pita and secure with toothpicks.

Nutrition Information:

- Calories: 290

- Protein: 25g

- Carbohydrates: 30g

- Fat: 10g

- Fiber: 5g

- Sugar: 4g

- Portion Size: 1 serving

Tomato Basil Soup with Whole Grain Croutons

Ingredients:

- Tomatoes, diced

- Onion, chopped

- Garlic, minced

- Vegetable broth

- Fresh basil, chopped

- Whole grain bread, cubed

- Olive oil

- Salt and pepper to taste

Instructions:

1. Sauté onion and garlic until softened.

2. Add diced tomatoes, vegetable broth, and fresh basil.

3. Simmer until tomatoes are cooked.

4. In a separate pan, toast whole grain bread cubes in olive oil.

5. Serve soup with whole grain croutons.

Nutrition Information:

- Calories: 180
- Protein: 5g
- Carbohydrates: 30g
- Fat: 5g
- Fiber: 6g
- Sugar: 10g
- Portion Size: 1 serving

Zucchini Noodles with Pesto and Cherry Tomatoes

Ingredients:

- Zucchini, spiralized
- Cherry tomatoes, halved
- Pesto sauce

- Parmesan cheese, grated

- Pine nuts, toasted

Instructions:

1. Spiralize zucchini into noodles.

2. Toss zucchini noodles with pesto sauce.

3. Top with cherry tomatoes, Parmesan cheese, and toasted pine nuts.

Nutrition Information:

- Calories: 220

- Protein: 8g

- Carbohydrates: 15g

- Fat: 18g

- Fiber: 4g

- Sugar: 5g

- Portion Size: 1 serving

Chapter 4: Dinner Recipes

These carefully curated recipes emphasize balance, flavor, and nutritional value, ensuring a satisfying dining experience while keeping pre-diabetes management in mind.

Baked Lemon Herb Chicken

Ingredients:

- 4 boneless, skinless chicken breasts
- 2 tablespoons olive oil
- 1 lemon (juiced)
- 2 cloves garlic (minced)
- 1 teaspoon dried thyme
- 1 teaspoon dried rosemary
- Salt and pepper to taste

Instructions:

1. Preheat the oven to 375°F (190°C).
2. In a bowl, mix olive oil, lemon juice, minced garlic, dried thyme, dried rosemary, salt, and pepper.

3. Place chicken breasts in a baking dish and pour the lemon herb mixture over them.

4. Bake for 25-30 minutes or until chicken is cooked through.

5. Serve hot.

Nutrition Information (per serving):

- Calories: 250

- Protein: 30g

- Carbohydrates: 2g

- Fat: 12g

- Fiber: 0.5g

- Sugar: 0.5g

- Portion size: 1 chicken breast

Spaghetti Squash with Turkey Bolognese

Ingredients:

- 1 medium spaghetti squash

- 1 lb ground turkey

- 1 onion (chopped)

- 2 cloves garlic (minced)
- 1 can (28 oz) crushed tomatoes
- 1 teaspoon dried oregano
- 1 teaspoon dried basil
- Salt and pepper to taste
- Fresh basil for garnish

Instructions:

1. Preheat the oven to 375°F (190°C).
2. Cut the spaghetti squash in half, scoop out seeds, and bake for 30-40 minutes.
3. In a skillet, cook ground turkey until browned. Add chopped onion and minced garlic.
4. Stir in crushed tomatoes, oregano, basil, salt, and pepper. Simmer for 15-20 minutes.
5. Scrape the spaghetti squash with a fork to create "noodles" and top with turkey bolognese.
6. Garnish with fresh basil.

Nutrition Information (per serving):

- Calories: 320
- Protein: 25g

- Carbohydrates: 30g

- Fat: 12g

- Fiber: 8g

- Sugar: 12g

- Portion size: 1 cup squash with turkey sauce

Grilled Vegetable and Quinoa Stuffed Bell Peppers

Ingredients:

- 4 bell peppers (halved and seeds removed)

- 1 cup quinoa (cooked)

- 1 zucchini (diced)

- 1 yellow squash (diced)

- 1 cup cherry tomatoes (halved)

- 1 cup spinach (chopped)

- 1/2 cup feta cheese (crumbled)

- 2 tablespoons olive oil

- 1 teaspoon dried thyme

- Salt and pepper to taste

Instructions:

1. Preheat the grill to medium-high heat.
2. In a bowl, mix quinoa, diced zucchini, diced yellow squash, cherry tomatoes, chopped spinach, feta cheese, olive oil, dried thyme, salt, and pepper.
3. Stuff each bell pepper half with the quinoa and vegetable mixture.
4. Grill for 10-15 minutes or until peppers are tender.
5. Serve warm.

Nutrition Information (per serving):

- Calories: 280
- Protein: 10g
- Carbohydrates: 35g
- Fat: 10g
- Fiber: 6g
- Sugar: 8g
- Portion size: 2 stuffed pepper halves

Teriyaki Salmon with Brown Rice

Ingredients:

- 4 salmon fillets

- 1/2 cup teriyaki sauce
- 2 tablespoons honey
- 1 tablespoon soy sauce
- 2 cups brown rice (cooked)
- Sesame seeds for garnish
- Green onions (sliced) for garnish

Instructions:

1. Preheat the oven to 400°F (200°C).
2. In a bowl, mix teriyaki sauce, honey, and soy sauce.
3. Place salmon fillets in a baking dish and pour the teriyaki mixture over them.
4. Bake for 15-20 minutes or until salmon is cooked through.
5. Serve over a bed of cooked brown rice, garnished with sesame seeds and sliced green onions.

Nutrition Information (per serving):

- Calories: 350
- Protein: 25g
- Carbohydrates: 40g
- Fat: 12g

- Fiber: 2g

- Sugar: 8g

- Portion size: 1 salmon fillet with rice

Cauliflower Crust Margherita Pizza

Ingredients:

- 1 cauliflower head (riced)

- 1 cup mozzarella cheese (shredded)

- 1 egg

- 1 teaspoon dried oregano

- 1/2 cup tomato sauce

- 1 large tomato (sliced)

- Fresh basil leaves

- Salt and pepper to taste

Instructions:

1. Preheat the oven to 425°F (220°C).

2. Microwave riced cauliflower for 5 minutes and squeeze out excess moisture using a kitchen towel.

3. In a bowl, mix cauliflower, mozzarella cheese, egg, dried oregano, salt, and pepper.

4. Press the cauliflower mixture onto a parchment-lined baking sheet to form a crust.

5. Bake for 15-20 minutes or until the crust is golden.

6. Spread tomato sauce over the crust, add sliced tomatoes, and bake for an additional 10 minutes.

7. Garnish with fresh basil leaves.

Nutrition Information (per serving):

- Calories: 200

- Protein: 10g

- Carbohydrates: 20g

- Fat: 10g

- Fiber: 5g

- Sugar: 6g

- Portion size: 2 slices

Blackened Tilapia with Quinoa Pilaf

Ingredients:

- 4 tilapia fillets

- 1 tablespoon paprika

- 1 teaspoon dried thyme

- 1 teaspoon garlic powder

- 1 teaspoon onion powder
- 1 teaspoon cayenne pepper
- 2 cups quinoa (cooked)
- 1 cup mixed vegetables (peas, carrots, corn)
- Lemon wedges for serving

Instructions:

1. In a bowl, mix paprika, dried thyme, garlic powder, onion powder, and cayenne pepper.
2. Coat tilapia fillets with the spice mixture.
3. Cook tilapia on a preheated skillet for 3-4 minutes per side or until blackened.
4. In a separate pan, sauté mixed vegetables and add cooked quinoa.
5. Serve blackened tilapia over quinoa pilaf with lemon wedges.

Nutrition Information (per serving):

- Calories: 280
- Protein: 25g
- Carbohydrates: 35g
- Fat: 6g

- Fiber: 5g

- Sugar: 2g

- Portion size: 1 tilapia fillet with quinoa

Turkey and Sweet Potato Skillet

Ingredients:

- 1 lb ground turkey

- 2 sweet potatoes (peeled and diced)

- 1 onion (chopped)

- 2 bell peppers (sliced)

- 2 tablespoons olive oil

- 1 teaspoon cumin

- 1 teaspoon smoked paprika

- Salt and pepper to taste

- Fresh cilantro for garnish

Instructions:

1. In a skillet, cook ground turkey until browned. Set aside.

2. In the same skillet, heat olive oil and sauté sweet potatoes until slightly tender.

3. Add chopped onion and sliced bell peppers. Cook until vegetables are soft.

4. Mix in the cooked turkey, cumin, smoked paprika, salt, and pepper.

5. Garnish with fresh cilantro before serving.

Nutrition Information (per serving):

- Calories: 320
- Protein: 20g
- Carbohydrates: 30g
- Fat: 15g
- Fiber: 6g
- Sugar: 8g
- Portion size: 1 cup

Eggplant Lasagna

Ingredients:

- 1 large eggplant (sliced)
- 1 lb ground beef or turkey
- 1 onion (chopped)
- 2 cloves garlic (minced)
- 2 cups marinara sauce

- 1 teaspoon dried oregano
- 1 teaspoon dried basil
- 2 cups ricotta cheese
- 2 cups mozzarella cheese (shredded)
- Salt and pepper to taste
- Fresh parsley for garnish

Instructions:

1. Preheat the oven to 375°F (190°C).
2. Grill or bake eggplant slices until tender.
3. In a skillet, cook ground beef or turkey until browned. Add chopped onion and minced garlic.
4. Stir in marinara sauce, dried oregano, and dried basil. Simmer for 10 minutes.
5. In a baking dish, layer eggplant slices, meat sauce, ricotta cheese, and mozzarella cheese.
6. Repeat the layers, finishing with a layer of mozzarella on top.
7. Bake for 30-35 minutes or until bubbly and golden.
8. Garnish with fresh parsley before serving.

Nutrition Information (per serving):

- Calories: 380
- Protein: 30g
- Carbohydrates: 20g
- Fat: 20g
- Fiber: 5g
- Sugar: 8g
- Portion size: 1 slice

Coconut Curry Chicken with Vegetables

Ingredients:

- 1 lb chicken breast (cubed)
- 1 cup broccoli florets
- 1 cup carrots (sliced)
- 1 bell pepper (sliced)
- 1 can (14 oz) coconut milk
- 2 tablespoons red curry paste
- 1 tablespoon soy sauce
- 1 tablespoon brown sugar
- 1 tablespoon vegetable oil

- Fresh cilantro for garnish

Instructions:

1. In a wok or large skillet, heat vegetable oil and sauté chicken until browned.
2. Add sliced carrots, broccoli florets, and bell pepper. Cook until vegetables are tender-crisp.
3. Stir in red curry paste, soy sauce, and brown sugar.
4. Pour in coconut milk and simmer until chicken is cooked through.
5. Garnish with fresh cilantro before serving.

Nutrition Information (per serving):

- Calories: 420
- Protein: 25g
- Carbohydrates: 15g
- Fat: 30g
- Fiber: 4g
- Sugar: 6g
- Portion size: 1 cup

Lemon Garlic Shrimp with Whole Wheat Pasta

Ingredients:

- 1 lb shrimp (peeled and deveined)
- 2 cups whole wheat pasta (cooked)
- 3 tablespoons olive oil
- 3 cloves garlic (minced)
- 1 lemon (zested and juiced)
- 1/2 teaspoon red pepper flakes
- Salt and pepper to taste
- Fresh parsley for garnish

Instructions:

1. In a pan, heat olive oil and sauté minced garlic until fragrant.
2. Add shrimp and cook until pink and opaque.
3. Toss in cooked whole wheat pasta, lemon zest, lemon juice, red pepper flakes, salt, and pepper.
4. Stir until well combined and heated through.
5. Garnish with fresh parsley before serving.

Nutrition Information (per serving):

- Calories: 350
- Protein: 20g
- Carbohydrates: 40g
- Fat: 12g
- Fiber: 6g
- Sugar: 2g
- Portion size: 1 cup

Stuffed Acorn Squash with Wild Rice

Ingredients:

- 2 acorn squashes (halved and seeds removed)
- 1 cup wild rice (cooked)
- 1 cup mushrooms (sliced)
- 1/2 cup dried cranberries
- 1/4 cup pecans (chopped)
- 2 tablespoons olive oil
- 1 teaspoon dried sage
- Salt and pepper to taste

Instructions:

1. Preheat the oven to 375°F (190°C).

2. Rub acorn squashes with olive oil and sprinkle with salt and pepper.

3. Roast squashes for 30-40 minutes or until tender.

4. In a pan, sauté mushrooms until browned. Mix with cooked wild rice, dried cranberries, chopped pecans, dried sage, salt, and pepper.

5. Stuff each acorn squash half with the wild rice mixture.

6. Serve warm.

Nutrition Information (per serving):

- Calories: 280
- Protein: 8g
- Carbohydrates: 45g
- Fat: 10g
- Fiber: 6g
- Sugar: 12g
- Portion size: 1 stuffed squash half

Ratatouille

Ingredients:

- 1 eggplant (sliced)

- 1 zucchini (sliced)
- 1 yellow squash (sliced)
- 1 bell pepper (sliced)
- 1 onion (sliced)
- 2 cloves garlic (minced)
- 1 can (14 oz) crushed tomatoes
- 1 teaspoon dried thyme
- 1 teaspoon dried rosemary
- 2 tablespoons olive oil
- Salt and pepper to taste

Instructions:

1. Preheat the oven to 375°F (190°C).
2. In a baking dish, layer sliced eggplant, zucchini, yellow squash, bell pepper, and onion.
3. Mix minced garlic, crushed tomatoes, dried thyme, dried rosemary, olive oil, salt, and pepper.
4. Pour the tomato mixture over the layered vegetables.
5. Bake for 45-50 minutes or until vegetables are tender.
6. Serve as a side or over whole wheat couscous.

Nutrition Information (per serving):

- Calories: 220
- Protein: 5g
- Carbohydrates: 35g
- Fat: 8g
- Fiber: 10g
- Sugar: 12g
- Portion size: 1 cup

Sesame Ginger Tofu Stir-Fry

Ingredients:

- 1 lb firm tofu (cubed)
- 2 cups broccoli florets
- 1 bell pepper (sliced)
- 1 carrot (julienned)
- 2 tablespoons soy sauce
- 1 tablespoon sesame oil
- 1 tablespoon rice vinegar
- 1 tablespoon honey
- 1 tablespoon ginger (minced)
- 2 cloves garlic (minced)
- Sesame seeds for garnish

- Green onions (sliced) for garnish

Instructions:

1. Press tofu to remove excess water and cut into cubes.

2. In a wok or skillet, stir-fry tofu until golden brown. Set aside.

3. In the same pan, stir-fry broccoli, bell pepper, and julienned carrot until crisp-tender.

4. Mix soy sauce, sesame oil, rice vinegar, honey, minced ginger, and minced garlic. Add to the vegetables.

5. Add the tofu back to the pan and toss until well coated.

6. Garnish with sesame seeds and sliced green onions.

Nutrition Information (per serving):

- Calories: 300
- Protein: 15g
- Carbohydrates: 25g
- Fat: 18g
- Fiber: 6g
- Sugar: 8g

- Portion size: 1 cup

Cilantro Lime Chicken with Brown Rice

Ingredients:

- 1 lb chicken thighs (boneless, skinless)
- 1 cup brown rice (cooked)
- 1/4 cup fresh cilantro (chopped)
- 2 limes (juiced and zested)
- 2 tablespoons olive oil
- 2 cloves garlic (minced)
- 1 teaspoon cumin
- Salt and pepper to taste
- Lime wedges for serving

Instructions:

1. In a bowl, mix olive oil, lime juice, lime zest, minced garlic, cumin, salt, and pepper.
2. Marinate chicken thighs in the mixture for at least 30 minutes.
3. Grill or pan-cook chicken until fully cooked.

4. Serve over a bed of cooked brown rice.

5. Garnish with chopped cilantro and lime wedges.

Nutrition Information (per serving):

- Calories: 350

- Protein: 20g

- Carbohydrates: 30g

- Fat: 15g

- Fiber: 3g

- Sugar: 2g

- Portion size: 1 chicken thigh with rice

Roasted Brussels Sprouts and Chicken Thighs

Ingredients:

- 4 chicken thighs (bone-in, skin-on)

- 1 lb Brussels sprouts (trimmed and halved)

- 2 tablespoons olive oil

- 1 teaspoon garlic powder

- 1 teaspoon onion powder

- 1 teaspoon smoked paprika

- Salt and pepper to taste
- Fresh thyme for garnish

Instructions:

1. Preheat the oven to 425°F (220°C).
2. In a bowl, toss Brussels sprouts with olive oil, garlic powder, onion powder, smoked paprika, salt, and pepper.
3. Place chicken thighs on a baking sheet, surround with Brussels sprouts.
4. Roast for 35-40 minutes or until chicken is crispy and Brussels sprouts are golden.
5. Garnish with fresh thyme before serving.

Nutrition Information (per serving):

- Calories: 400
- Protein: 25g
- Carbohydrates: 15g
- Fat: 30g
- Fiber: 8g
- Sugar: 2g
- Portion size: 1 chicken thigh with Brussels sprouts

Chapter 5: Snacks and Appetizers

In this chapter, we present a collection of Snacks and Appetizers that not only tantalize your taste buds but also align with the principles of a balanced pre-diabetes-friendly diet. Let's dive into these delicious and health-conscious snack ideas.

Guacamole with Veggie Sticks

Ingredients:

- 2 ripe avocados
- 1 tomato, diced
- 1/4 cup red onion, finely chopped
- 1 clove garlic, minced
- 1 lime, juiced
- Salt and pepper to taste
- Veggie sticks (carrots, celery, bell peppers)

Instructions:

1. Mash avocados in a bowl.

2. Add diced tomatoes, chopped red onion, minced garlic, and lime juice. Mix well.
3. Season with salt and pepper to taste.
4. Serve with an assortment of veggie sticks.

Nutrition Information:

- Calories: 120
- Protein: 2g
- Carbohydrates: 10g
- Fat: 9g
- Fiber: 5g
- Sugar: 2g
- Portion Size: 1/4 cup guacamole with veggie sticks

Hummus and Whole Wheat Pita

Ingredients:

- 1 can chickpeas, drained
- 2 tablespoons tahini
- 2 cloves garlic
- 1 lemon, juiced
- 2 tablespoons olive oil
- Salt to taste

- Whole wheat pita, cut into triangles

Instructions:

1. Blend chickpeas, tahini, garlic, lemon juice, and olive oil until smooth.
2. Season with salt to taste.
3. Serve with whole wheat pita triangles.

Nutrition Information:

- Calories: 150
- Protein: 4g
- Carbohydrates: 20g
- Fat: 7g
- Fiber: 5g
- Sugar: 1g
- Portion Size: 2 tablespoons hummus with whole wheat pita

Greek Yogurt with Berries

Ingredients:

- 1 cup Greek yogurt
- Mixed berries (strawberries, blueberries, raspberries)

- Honey (optional for sweetness)

Instructions:

1. Spoon Greek yogurt into a bowl.
2. Top with mixed berries.
3. Drizzle with honey if desired.

Nutrition Information:

- Calories: 180
- Protein: 15g
- Carbohydrates: 20g
- Fat: 5g
- Fiber: 3g
- Sugar: 15g
- Portion Size: 1 cup Greek yogurt with berries

Roasted Chickpeas

Ingredients:

- 1 can chickpeas, drained and rinsed
- 1 tablespoon olive oil
- 1 teaspoon cumin
- 1 teaspoon paprika

- Salt to taste

Instructions:

1. Preheat oven to 400°F (200°C).
2. Toss chickpeas with olive oil, cumin, paprika, and salt.
3. Spread chickpeas on a baking sheet and roast for 25-30 minutes until crispy.

Nutrition Information:

- Calories: 160
- Protein: 5g
- Carbohydrates: 25g
- Fat: 5g
- Fiber: 5g
- Sugar: 5g
- Portion Size: 1/2 cup roasted chickpeas

Cottage Cheese and Pineapple

Ingredients:

- 1 cup low-fat cottage cheese
- Fresh pineapple chunks

Instructions:

1. Spoon cottage cheese into a bowl.
2. Top with fresh pineapple chunks.

Nutrition Information:

- Calories: 200
- Protein: 20g
- Carbohydrates: 25g
- Fat: 2g
- Fiber: 2g
- Sugar: 15g
- Portion Size: 1 cup cottage cheese with pineapple

Caprese Skewers

Ingredients:

- Cherry tomatoes
- Fresh mozzarella balls
- Fresh basil leaves
- Balsamic glaze for drizzling

Instructions:

1. Thread a tomato, mozzarella ball, and basil leaf onto small skewers.

2. Arrange on a serving platter and drizzle with balsamic glaze.

Nutrition Information:

- Calories: 120
- Protein: 8g
- Carbohydrates: 5g
- Fat: 8g
- Fiber: 1g
- Sugar: 2g
- Portion Size: 3 skewers

Trail Mix with Nuts and Dried Fruit

Ingredients:

- 1/2 cup almonds
- 1/2 cup walnuts
- 1/4 cup dried cranberries
- 1/4 cup raisins
- 1/4 cup dark chocolate chips

Instructions:

1. Mix almonds, walnuts, dried cranberries, raisins, and dark chocolate chips in a bowl.
2. Portion into small snack-sized bags for easy grab-and-go.

Nutrition Information:

- Calories: 250
- Protein: 7g
- Carbohydrates: 20g
- Fat: 18g
- Fiber: 4g
- Sugar: 12g
- Portion Size: 1/2 cup trail mix

Sliced Apple with Almond Butter

Ingredients:

- 1 apple, sliced
- 2 tablespoons almond butter

Instructions:

1. Arrange apple slices on a plate.

2. Dip each slice into almond butter before eating.

Nutrition Information:

- Calories: 180
- Protein: 3g
- Carbohydrates: 25g
- Fat: 8g
- Fiber: 5g
- Sugar: 18g
- Portion Size: 1 sliced apple with almond butter

Baked Sweet Potato Fries

Ingredients:

- 2 sweet potatoes, cut into fries
- 1 tablespoon olive oil
- 1 teaspoon paprika
- Salt and pepper to taste

Instructions:

1. Preheat oven to 425°F (220°C).
2. Toss sweet potato fries with olive oil, paprika, salt, and pepper.

3. Bake for 25-30 minutes until crispy.

Nutrition Information:

- Calories: 160
- Protein: 2g
- Carbohydrates: 30g
- Fat: 4g
- Fiber: 5g
- Sugar: 6g
- Portion Size: 1 cup baked sweet potato fries

Edamame with Sea Salt

Ingredients:

- 1 cup edamame (unshelled)
- Sea salt for sprinkling

Instructions:

1. Steam or boil edamame until tender.
2. Sprinkle with sea salt before serving.

Nutrition Information:

- Calories: 120

- Protein: 11g
- Carbohydrates: 10g
- Fat: 5g
- Fiber: 5g
- Sugar: 3g
- Portion Size: 1 cup edamame with sea salt

Cucumber and Feta Bites

Ingredients:

- English cucumber, sliced
- Feta cheese, crumbled
- Cherry tomatoes, halved
- Fresh mint leaves
- Balsamic glaze for drizzling

Instructions:

1. Place cucumber slices on a serving platter.
2. Top each slice with crumbled feta, halved cherry tomatoes, and a mint leaf.
3. Drizzle with balsamic glaze before serving.

Nutrition Information:

- Calories: 90
- Protein: 4g
- Carbohydrates: 5g
- Fat: 6g
- Fiber: 1g
- Sugar: 3g
- Portion Size: 5 cucumber and feta bites

Greek Hummus Dip

Ingredients:

- 1 cup hummus
- 1 tablespoon olive oil
- 1 teaspoon dried oregano
- Kalamata olives for garnish
- Whole grain tortilla chips for dipping

Instructions:

1. Spread hummus on a serving plate.
2. Drizzle with olive oil and sprinkle dried oregano.
3. Garnish with Kalamata olives.
4. Serve with whole grain tortilla chips.

Nutrition Information:

- Calories: 180
- Protein: 5g
- Carbohydrates: 20g
- Fat: 10g
- Fiber: 5g
- Sugar: 2g
- Portion Size: 2 tablespoons hummus with tortilla chips

Almond and Cranberry Energy Balls

Ingredients:

- 1 cup almonds
- 1/2 cup dried cranberries
- 1/4 cup almond butter
- 1/4 cup honey
- 1/2 teaspoon vanilla extract

Instructions:

1. Blend almonds and dried cranberries in a food processor.

2. Add almond butter, honey, and vanilla extract. Pulse until well combined.

3. Roll mixture into small energy balls.

Nutrition Information:

- Calories: 120
- Protein: 3g
- Carbohydrates: 15g
- Fat: 7g
- Fiber: 2g
- Sugar: 10g
- Portion Size: 2 energy balls

Salsa and Whole Grain Tortilla Chips

Ingredients:

- 1 cup fresh salsa
- Whole grain tortilla chips

Instructions:

1. Pour fresh salsa into a bowl.
2. Serve with whole grain tortilla chips.

Nutrition Information:

- Calories: 140
- Protein: 3g
- Carbohydrates: 20g
- Fat: 5g
- Fiber: 3g
- Sugar: 5g
- Portion Size: 1/2 cup salsa with tortilla chips

Stuffed Mini Bell Peppers with Goat Cheese

Ingredients:

- Mini bell peppers, halved and deseeded
- Goat cheese
- Fresh parsley, chopped for garnish

Instructions:

1. Fill each mini bell pepper half with goat cheese.
2. Garnish with fresh parsley before serving.

Nutrition Information:

- Calories: 110
- Protein: 5g
- Carbohydrates: 8g
- Fat: 7g
- Fiber: 2g
- Sugar: 5g
- Portion Size: 5 stuffed mini bell peppers

Chapter 6: Desserts

This chapter is a treasure trove of sweet treats designed to satiate your cravings while keeping your health in mind. From refreshing popsicles to rich chocolate truffles, each recipe is carefully crafted to balance flavor and nutrition.

Mixed Berry Parfait

Ingredients:

- 1 cup mixed berries (strawberries, blueberries, raspberries)
- 1 cup Greek yogurt (unsweetened)
- 2 tablespoons honey
- 1/4 cup granola (optional)

Instructions:

1. In a glass or bowl, layer mixed berries.
2. Top with a dollop of Greek yogurt.
3. Drizzle honey over the yogurt.
4. Repeat the layers.
5. Finish with a sprinkle of granola if desired.

Nutrition Information:

- Calories: 200
- Protein: 8g
- Carbohydrates: 30g
- Fat: 6g
- Fiber: 5g
- Sugar: 18g
- Portion Size: 1 serving

Dark Chocolate-Dipped Strawberries

Ingredients:

- 1 cup dark chocolate chips (70% cocoa or higher)
- 1 pint fresh strawberries, washed and dried

Instructions:

1. Melt the dark chocolate in a heatproof bowl.
2. Dip each strawberry into the melted chocolate, covering half.
3. Place on parchment paper and let it cool until the chocolate hardens.

Nutrition Information:

- Calories: 120
- Protein: 2g
- Carbohydrates: 15g
- Fat: 7g
- Fiber: 4g
- Sugar: 8g
- Portion Size: 4 strawberries

Greek Yogurt and Honey Popsicles

Ingredients:

- 2 cups Greek yogurt (unsweetened)
- 1/4 cup honey
- 1 teaspoon vanilla extract

Instructions:

1. In a bowl, mix Greek yogurt, honey, and vanilla extract.
2. Pour the mixture into popsicle molds.
3. Freeze for at least 4 hours.

Nutrition Information:

- Calories: 150
- Protein: 10g
- Carbohydrates: 20g
- Fat: 5g
- Fiber: 1g
- Sugar: 15g
- Portion Size: 1 popsicle

Baked Apple with Cinnamon

Ingredients:

- 2 medium-sized apples
- 1 teaspoon cinnamon
- 1 tablespoon chopped almonds

Instructions:

1. Core the apples and place them in a baking dish.
2. Sprinkle cinnamon over the apples.
3. Bake at 350°F (180°C) for 20-25 minutes.
4. Top with chopped almonds before serving.

Nutrition Information:

- Calories: 180
- Protein: 2g
- Carbohydrates: 40g
- Fat: 3g
- Fiber: 7g
- Sugar: 28g
- Portion Size: 1 apple

Berry and Almond Crisp

Ingredients:

- 2 cups mixed berries (strawberries, blueberries, blackberries)
- 1/2 cup almond flour
- 1/4 cup rolled oats
- 2 tablespoons honey
- 2 tablespoons melted coconut oil
- 1/4 cup sliced almonds

Instructions:

1. Preheat the oven to 350°F (180°C).

2. In a bowl, mix berries with honey and place in a baking dish.

3. In another bowl, combine almond flour, oats, melted coconut oil, and sliced almonds.

4. Sprinkle the almond mixture over the berries.

5. Bake for 25-30 minutes or until the top is golden brown.

Nutrition Information:

- Calories: 220
- Protein: 5g
- Carbohydrates: 30g
- Fat: 10g
- Fiber: 6g
- Sugar: 15g
- Portion Size: 1 serving

Avocado Chocolate Mousse

Ingredients:

- 2 ripe avocados
- 1/4 cup unsweetened cocoa powder
- 1/4 cup honey

- 1 teaspoon vanilla extract
- Pinch of salt

Instructions:

1. Blend avocados, cocoa powder, honey, vanilla extract, and salt until smooth.
2. Chill in the refrigerator for at least 1 hour before serving.

Nutrition Information:

- Calories: 180
- Protein: 3g
- Carbohydrates: 20g
- Fat: 12g
- Fiber: 7g
- Sugar: 10g
- Portion Size: 1/2 cup

Pumpkin Pie Chia Pudding

Ingredients:

- 1/4 cup chia seeds
- 1 cup unsweetened almond milk

- 1/2 cup canned pumpkin puree
- 1 tablespoon maple syrup
- 1/2 teaspoon pumpkin pie spice

Instructions:

1. In a bowl, mix chia seeds, almond milk, pumpkin puree, maple syrup, and pumpkin pie spice.
2. Refrigerate for at least 2 hours or overnight.

Nutrition Information:

- Calories: 120
- Protein: 4g
- Carbohydrates: 15g
- Fat: 6g
- Fiber: 8g
- Sugar: 5g
- Portion Size: 1/2 cup

Coconut and Berry Sorbet

Ingredients:

- 2 cups mixed berries (strawberries, blueberries, raspberries)

- 1 can (14 oz) coconut milk
- 1/4 cup honey
- Juice of 1 lime

Instructions:

1. Blend berries, coconut milk, honey, and lime juice until smooth.
2. Pour the mixture into an ice cream maker and churn according to the manufacturer's instructions.
3. Freeze for an additional 2 hours before serving.

Nutrition Information:

- Calories: 160
- Protein: 2g
- Carbohydrates: 20g
- Fat: 9g
- Fiber: 4g
- Sugar: 14g
- Portion Size: 1/2 cup

Almond Flour Banana Bread

Ingredients:

- 2 ripe bananas, mashed
- 3 eggs
- 1/4 cup coconut oil, melted
- 1 teaspoon vanilla extract
- 2 cups almond flour
- 1 teaspoon baking soda
- Pinch of salt

Instructions:

1. Preheat the oven to 350°F (180°C).
2. In a bowl, mix mashed bananas, eggs, melted coconut oil, and vanilla extract.
3. Add almond flour, baking soda, and salt. Mix until well combined.
4. Pour the batter into a greased loaf pan and bake for 40-45 minutes.

Nutrition Information:

- Calories: 200
- Protein: 6g

- Carbohydrates: 15g

- Fat: 14g

- Fiber: 4g

- Sugar: 8g

- Portion Size: 1 slice

Mango and Yogurt Frozen Bites

Ingredients:

- 1 cup diced mango

- 1 cup Greek yogurt (unsweetened)

- 2 tablespoons honey

Instructions:

1. In a blender, puree diced mango until smooth.

2. In a bowl, mix Greek yogurt and honey.

3. Layer mango puree and yogurt mixture in ice cube trays.

4. Freeze for at least 3 hours.

Nutrition Information:

- Calories: 80

- Protein: 3g

- Carbohydrates: 15g
- Fat: 1g
- Fiber: 1g
- Sugar: 12g
- Portion Size: 2 bites

Chocolate Avocado Truffles

Ingredients:

- 2 ripe avocados
- 1/2 cup unsweetened cocoa powder
- 1/4 cup maple syrup
- 1 teaspoon vanilla extract
- 1/4 cup shredded coconut (optional)

Instructions:

1. In a food processor, blend avocados, cocoa powder, maple syrup, and vanilla extract until smooth.
2. Roll the mixture into small truffle-sized balls.
3. Optional: Roll truffles in shredded coconut.
4. Refrigerate for at least 1 hour before serving.

Nutrition Information:

- Calories: 90
- Protein: 2g
- Carbohydrates: 10g
- Fat: 6g
- Fiber: 4g
- Sugar: 4g
- Portion Size: 2 truffles

Lemon Blueberry Yogurt Cake

Ingredients:

- 1 cup almond flour
- 1/2 cup coconut flour
- 1 teaspoon baking powder
- 1/2 teaspoon baking soda
- Pinch of salt
- 3 eggs
- 1/4 cup coconut oil, melted
- 1/4 cup honey
- 1 cup Greek yogurt (unsweetened)
- 1 teaspoon vanilla extract
- Zest of 1 lemon

- 1 cup blueberries

Instructions:

1. Preheat the oven to 350°F (180°C).
2. In a bowl, whisk almond flour, coconut flour, baking powder, baking soda, and salt.
3. In another bowl, whisk eggs, melted coconut oil, honey, Greek yogurt, vanilla extract, and lemon zest.
4. Combine wet and dry ingredients. Fold in blueberries.
5. Pour the batter into a greased cake pan and bake for 30-35 minutes.

Nutrition Information:

- Calories: 220
- Protein: 7g
- Carbohydrates: 20g
- Fat: 14g
- Fiber: 5g
- Sugar: 10g
- Portion Size: 1 slice

Strawberry Shortcake Cups

Ingredients:

- 2 cups sliced strawberries
- 1 cup almond flour
- 1/4 cup coconut flour
- 1 teaspoon baking powder
- 1/4 teaspoon salt
- 3 tablespoons coconut oil, melted
- 3 tablespoons honey
- 1 teaspoon vanilla extract
- Greek yogurt (unsweetened) for topping

Instructions:

1. Preheat the oven to 350°F (180°C).
2. In a bowl, combine almond flour, coconut flour, baking powder, and salt.
3. In another bowl, mix melted coconut oil, honey, and vanilla extract.
4. Combine wet and dry ingredients to form a dough.
5. Press the dough into muffin cups to create cups.
6. Bake for 12-15 minutes. Let them cool.

7. Fill each cup with sliced strawberries and top with a dollop of Greek yogurt.

Nutrition Information:

- Calories: 180
- Protein: 4g
- Carbohydrates: 18g
- Fat: 10g
- Fiber: 4g
- Sugar: 10g
- Portion Size: 2 cups

Pistachio and Cranberry Bark

Ingredients:

- 1 cup dark chocolate chips (70% cocoa or higher)
- 1/4 cup shelled pistachios, chopped
- 1/4 cup dried cranberries

Instructions:

1. Melt the dark chocolate in a heatproof bowl.
2. Mix in chopped pistachios and dried cranberries.
3. Spread the mixture on a parchment paper-lined tray.

4. Allow it to cool and harden before breaking it into
   pieces.

Nutrition Information:

- Calories: 160
- Protein: 3g
- Carbohydrates: 20g
- Fat: 9g
- Fiber: 4g
- Sugar: 12g
- Portion Size: 1/4 cup

Raspberry and Almond Chia Seed Pudding

Ingredients:

- 1/4 cup chia seeds
- 1 cup unsweetened almond milk
- 1/2 cup fresh raspberries
- 1 tablespoon almond butter
- 1 tablespoon honey

Instructions:

1. In a jar, mix chia seeds and almond milk. Refrigerate for at least 2 hours.

2. In a blender, puree raspberries, almond butter, and honey.

3. Layer chia pudding and raspberry puree in serving glasses.

Nutrition Information:

- Calories: 180
- Protein: 5g
- Carbohydrates: 20g
- Fat: 10g
- Fiber: 9g
- Sugar: 8g
- Portion Size: 1 serving

Chapter 7: Smoothies

In this chapter, we present a collection of smoothie recipes designed to tantalize your taste buds while providing essential nutrients. These smoothies are not only a treat for your palate but also a nourishing addition to your Pre-Diabetes Diet Plan.

Green Goddess Smoothie

Ingredients:

- 1 cup fresh spinach leaves
- 1/2 ripe avocado
- 1/2 cucumber, peeled and sliced
- 1 green apple, cored and chopped
- 1 cup almond milk
- Ice cubes (optional)

Instructions:

1. Combine all ingredients in a blender.
2. Blend until smooth and creamy.
3. Pour into a glass and enjoy!

Nutrition Information (per serving):

- Calories: 180
- Protein: 5g
- Carbohydrates: 20g
- Fat: 10g
- Fiber: 7g
- Sugar: 10g
- Portion size: 1 serving

Berry Blast Smoothie

Ingredients:

- 1 cup mixed berries (strawberries, blueberries, raspberries)
- 1/2 banana
- 1/2 cup Greek yogurt
- 1 cup unsweetened almond milk
- 1 tablespoon honey (optional)

Instructions:

1. Combine berries, banana, Greek yogurt, and almond milk in a blender.
2. Blend until smooth.

3. Add honey if desired, blend again.

4. Pour into a glass and savor the berry goodness!

Nutrition Information (per serving):

- Calories: 220

- Protein: 8g

- Carbohydrates: 35g

- Fat: 5g

- Fiber: 6g

- Sugar: 25g

- Portion size: 1 serving

Tropical Paradise Smoothie

Ingredients:

- 1/2 cup pineapple chunks

- 1/2 cup mango chunks

- 1/2 banana

- 1/2 cup coconut milk

- Ice cubes (optional)

Instructions:

1. Blend pineapple, mango, banana, and coconut milk until smooth.
2. Add ice cubes if a colder consistency is desired.
3. Pour into a glass and transport yourself to a tropical paradise!

Nutrition Information (per serving):

*   Calories: 200
*   Protein: 4g
*   Carbohydrates: 40g
*   Fat: 6g
*   Fiber: 5g
*   Sugar: 25g
*   Portion size: 1 serving

Peanut Butter Banana Smoothie

Ingredients:

*   1 ripe banana
*   2 tablespoons peanut butter
*   1 cup unsweetened almond milk
*   1 tablespoon chia seeds

- Ice cubes (optional)

Instructions:

1. Blend banana, peanut butter, almond milk, and chia
   seeds until smooth.
2. Add ice cubes if desired.
3. Pour into a glass and relish the creamy goodness.

Nutrition Information (per serving):

- Calories: 250
- Protein: 8g
- Carbohydrates: 20g
- Fat: 15g
- Fiber: 6g
- Sugar: 8g
- Portion size: 1 serving

Spinach and Pineapple Smoothie

Ingredients:

- 1 cup fresh spinach leaves
- 1 cup pineapple chunks
- 1/2 banana

- 1/2 cup Greek yogurt

- 1/2 cup water

Instructions:

1. Blend spinach, pineapple, banana, Greek yogurt, and water until smooth.

2. Pour into a glass and enjoy this nutrient-packed green delight!

Nutrition Information (per serving):

- Calories: 180

- Protein: 6g

- Carbohydrates: 30g

- Fat: 3g

- Fiber: 5g

- Sugar: 18g

- Portion size: 1 serving

Mango and Coconut Smoothie

Ingredients:

- 1 cup mango chunks

- 1/2 cup coconut milk

- 1/2 cup Greek yogurt
- 1 tablespoon honey
- Ice cubes (optional)

Instructions:

1. Blend mango, coconut milk, Greek yogurt, and honey until smooth.
2. Add ice cubes for a refreshing twist.
3. Pour into a glass and savor the tropical fusion!

Nutrition Information (per serving):

- Calories: 220
- Protein: 7g
- Carbohydrates: 35g
- Fat: 6g
- Fiber: 4g
- Sugar: 28g
- Portion size: 1 serving

Blueberry Almond Smoothie

Ingredients:

- 1 cup blueberries

- 1/4 cup almonds
- 1/2 banana
- 1 cup almond milk
- Ice cubes (optional)

Instructions:

1. Blend blueberries, almonds, banana, and almond milk until smooth.
2. Add ice cubes for a chilled consistency.
3. Pour into a glass and indulge in the antioxidant-rich blend.

Nutrition Information (per serving):

- Calories: 230
- Protein: 6g
- Carbohydrates: 30g
- Fat: 11g
- Fiber: 7g
- Sugar: 15g
- Portion size: 1 serving

Kale and Kiwi Smoothie

Ingredients:

- 1 cup kale leaves, stems removed
- 2 kiwis, peeled and sliced
- 1/2 cup pineapple chunks
- 1/2 cup coconut water
- Ice cubes (optional)

Instructions:

1. Blend kale, kiwi, pineapple, and coconut water until smooth.
2. Incorporate ice cubes if a colder temperature is preferred.
3. Pour into a glass and revel in the vibrant green goodness.

Nutrition Information (per serving):

- Calories: 160
- Protein: 5g
- Carbohydrates: 35g
- Fat: 2g
- Fiber: 7g

- Sugar: 20g

- Portion size: 1 serving

Chocolate Protein Smoothie

Ingredients:

- 1 scoop chocolate protein powder

- 1 banana

- 1 tablespoon almond butter

- 1 cup almond milk

- Ice cubes (optional)

Instructions:

1. Blend chocolate protein powder, banana, almond butter, and almond milk until smooth.

2. Include ice cubes for a thicker texture.

3. Pour into a glass and relish the protein-packed chocolate delight.

Nutrition Information (per serving):

- Calories: 280

- Protein: 20g

- Carbohydrates: 30g

- Fat: 10g

- Fiber: 5g

- Sugar: 15g

- Portion size: 1 serving

Cucumber Mint Smoothie

Ingredients:

- 1/2 cucumber, peeled and sliced

- 1/2 cup fresh mint leaves

- 1/2 green apple, cored and chopped

- 1/2 cup plain Greek yogurt

- 1/2 cup water

Instructions:

1. Blend cucumber, mint, apple, Greek yogurt, and water until smooth.

2. Adjust the consistency with additional water if needed.

3. Pour into a glass and refresh your senses with this cooling blend.

Nutrition Information (per serving):

- Calories: 150

- Protein: 6g

- Carbohydrates: 25g

- Fat: 2g

- Fiber: 5g

- Sugar: 15g

- Portion size: 1 serving

Peach and Oat Smoothie

Ingredients:

- 1 cup sliced peaches (fresh or frozen)

- 1/4 cup rolled oats

- 1/2 banana

- 1 cup almond milk

- Ice cubes (optional)

Instructions:

1. Blend peaches, oats, banana, and almond milk until smooth.

2. Incorporate ice cubes for a colder texture.

3. Pour into a glass and relish the delightful combination of peaches and oats.

Nutrition Information (per serving):

- Calories: 210
- Protein: 5g
- Carbohydrates: 40g
- Fat: 4g
- Fiber: 6g
- Sugar: 18g
- Portion size: 1 serving

Acai Berry Smoothie Bowl

Ingredients:

- 1 pack frozen acai berry puree
- 1/2 cup mixed berries (strawberries, blueberries, raspberries)
- 1/2 banana
- 1/4 cup granola
- 1/4 cup coconut flakes

Instructions:

1. Blend acai puree, mixed berries, and banana until thick and smooth.

2. Pour into a bowl and top with granola and coconut flakes.

3. Enjoy this vibrant Acai Berry Smoothie Bowl with a spoon!

Nutrition Information (per serving):

- Calories: 280
- Protein: 6g
- Carbohydrates: 40g
- Fat: 12g
- Fiber: 8g
- Sugar: 18g
- Portion size: 1 serving

Watermelon Mint Smoothie

Ingredients:

- 2 cups diced watermelon
- 1/4 cup fresh mint leaves
- 1/2 lime, juiced

- 1/2 cup coconut water
- Ice cubes (optional)

Instructions:

1. Blend watermelon, mint, lime juice, and coconut water until smooth.
2. Add ice cubes for a refreshing chill.
3. Pour into a glass and relish the hydrating Watermelon Mint sensation.

Nutrition Information (per serving):

- Calories: 120
- Protein: 2g
- Carbohydrates: 30g
- Fat: 0g
- Fiber: 2g
- Sugar: 22g
- Portion size: 1 serving

Carrot Cake Smoothie

Ingredients:

- 1 cup shredded carrots

- 1/2 banana
- 1/4 cup walnuts
- 1 teaspoon cinnamon
- 1 cup almond milk
- Ice cubes (optional)

Instructions:

1. Blend shredded carrots, banana, walnuts, cinnamon, and almond milk until smooth.
2. Add ice cubes for a colder treat.
3. Pour into a glass and enjoy the taste of carrot cake in a liquid form.

Nutrition Information (per serving):

- Calories: 230
- Protein: 6g
- Carbohydrates: 25g
- Fat: 14g
- Fiber: 5g
- Sugar: 12g
- Portion size: 1 serving

Raspberry Avocado Smoothie

Ingredients:

- 1/2 cup fresh or frozen raspberries
- 1/2 ripe avocado
- 1/2 cup Greek yogurt
- 1 tablespoon honey
- 1 cup almond milk

Instructions:

1. Blend raspberries, avocado, Greek yogurt, honey, and almond milk until smooth.
2. Pour into a glass and savor the unique combination of raspberry and creamy avocado.

Nutrition Information (per serving):

- Calories: 220
- Protein: 7g
- Carbohydrates: 30g
- Fat: 10g
- Fiber: 8g
- Sugar: 18g
- Portion size: 1 serving

CONCLUSION

As we wrap up this Pre-Diabetes Diet Plan and Recipe Book, it's essential to reflect on the journey you're about to embark on. This isn't just a collection of recipes; it's a guide to transforming your lifestyle, fostering a healthier relationship with food, and taking charge of your well-being.

In the pages that precede this conclusion, we've meticulously crafted a 30-day meal plan, offering a varied selection of nutrient-dense and delectable dishes. From wholesome breakfasts to satisfying dinners, each recipe is designed not just to manage pre-diabetes but to elevate your culinary experience.

Beyond the vibrant flavors and appealing textures lies a deeper commitment to your health. We've delved into the intricacies of balancing nutrients, mastering portion control, and embracing a diverse array of ingredients. The journey towards a healthier you involves not just what you eat but how you approach food – as a source of nourishment, energy, and joy.

As you navigate the chapters, you'll find that this book extends beyond a mere cookbook. It's a comprehensive guide that encourages mindful eating, providing tips and insights to empower your choices. Remember, this is your journey, and you are in control. Take the time to savor the flavors, appreciate the colors on your plate, and relish the satisfaction of nourishing your body.

The recipes included aren't just about restriction; they're about discovery. Whether you're trying a new grain, exploring creative ways to incorporate vegetables, or blending exotic smoothie combinations, each recipe invites you to expand your culinary horizons.

In the realm of snacks, desserts, and smoothies, we've demonstrated that treating yourself doesn't have to compromise your health goals. Indulge sensibly, embrace the richness of natural flavors, and savor the sweetness of fruits and wholesome ingredients.

This book is a companion on your journey, offering guidance, inspiration, and a celebration of the joy that comes from mindful and health-conscious eating. Remember, small changes lead to significant results. With determination, commitment, and the culinary delights within these pages, you're not just managing pre-diabetes; you're crafting a lifestyle that honors your health and well-being.

May this book be a source of inspiration and encouragement as you embark on this transformative path. Here's to a future filled with vitality, flavorful meals, and the profound satisfaction of knowing you've taken the first steps towards a healthier, happier you. Cheers to your well-being!